Anti-aging Skincare Tips for Juniors

Unlocking the Secrets to Youthful Skin

Dr. Magdalene Wise

Copyright

1

As we age, our skin begins to alter, such as losing its suppleness and acquiring fine lines and wrinkles. While there is no way to halt time, developing a solid anti-aging skincare routine can help improve the appearance of any skin troubles.

What Exactly Are Wrinkles?

Wrinkles are creases and lines that appear on your skin. They are most commonly found on the face and neck, particularly around the eyes and lips, but they can arise elsewhere on the body. As we get older, our skin loses its elasticity and capacity to bounce back, making it more prone to wrinkles. Wrinkles are caused by several circumstances, including:

1. Aging: As previously said, the primary cause of wrinkles is aging. The skin produces less collagen and elastin, the proteins responsible for the skin's suppleness and firmness, throughout time.

2. Sun Exposure: Prolonged exposure to UltraViolet (UV) light from the sun is a key cause of premature skin aging and wrinkle formation. UV radiation can cause collagen and elastin fibres to break down, resulting in skin sagging and wrinkling.

3. Tobacco use degrades collagen and elastin, hastening the aging process and causing wrinkles to emerge earlier.

4. Facial Expressions: Repeated facial motions, such as smiling, frowning, or squinting, can cause dynamic wrinkles to appear. These creases are known as

"expression lines," and they become more noticeable over time.

5. Genetics: Some people are predisposed genetically to develop wrinkles early or more visibly than others.

6. Environmental Factors: Pollutants, free radicals, and exposure to extreme weather conditions can all contribute to skin damage and wrinkles.

There are various sorts of wrinkles, that include

- Fine Lines: The earliest and shallowest wrinkles, which are often scarcely visible. They usually appear around the eyes and mouth.

- Deep Lines: These are more noticeable and come from greater collagen and elastin loss.

- Wrinkles on the Neck and Chest: Wrinkles on the neck and chest are also common, especially due to sun exposure.

- Crow's Feet: Fine lines and wrinkles in the under-eye area, often known as crow's feet, are a good indicator of one's age. This is because the fragile skin around the eyes is generally the first to exhibit signs of ageing. Crow's feet wrinkles are an unavoidable aspect of ageing for many individuals, but they don't have to be your fate if you use the right skin care components and take the necessary precautions.

The Most Common Reasons for Forehead Wrinkles

Wrinkles can result from a variety of circumstances, including natural skin motions and excessive sun exposure. Check out these frequent causes of forehead wrinkles to learn more about how to avoid them.

Aging

It is common and natural to get wrinkles as you age. Skin cells divide more slowly as you age, and your skin thins as your connective tissue — elastin and collagen fibres — loosens.

Facial Movements That Are Repeated

Normal facial motions and expressions such as smiling, squinting, frowning, and wrinkling your brow or nose can accentuate fine lines and wrinkles.

Exposure to UV

Wrinkles and creases can form when UV light from the sun degrades your skin's collagen. It's one of the reasons we recommend wearing SPF every day, all year.

Tobacco Use

Cigarette smoking hastens the ageing process and reduces collagen formation. This, in turn, can cause wrinkles and thin lines to appear on the skin.

Once a wrinkle has formed, it is impossible to remove it without consulting a dermatologist and undergoing treatment with injectables or surgery. There are, however, various skincare and lifestyle modifications you can make to reduce their appearance, as well as activities you may take that will prevent wrinkles from forming in the first place.

Want to know how? Let's Go!

Different skin types

The first step in developing an effective skin care programme is determining your skin type. Assess the skin's appearance and texture, as well as how it reacts to cosmetics.

Normal Skin

Normal skin is clear and usually not sensitive to cosmetics. If the skin is drier during particular seasons, a lotion-based moisturiser may be used. A cream-based moisturiser may be more acceptable for menopausal women or anyone over the age of 50.

Sensitive Skin

People with sensitive skin should use products that are fragrance-free and designed for sensitive skin, such as cleansers and moisturisers. Anyone with rosacea, atopic dermatitis, also known as eczema, or allergy is likely to have a sensitive skin. To test for a reaction (commonly known as 'Patch Test'), apply a small amount to an area such as the inner forearm twice a day for 7-10 days. If the substance does not induce swelling, irritation, or other negative effects, it may be safe to use on a larger scale. If itching, a rash, or any response occurs, immediately wash the cream off and discontinue use.

Note Patch testing may not help those with rosacea because the ailment only affects the face.

Organic skin care products should be avoided by people with sensitive skin because some natural substances, such as essential oils, may irritate the skin.

Combination Skin

Combination skin indicates that some parts of the face are dry while others are oily, most commonly the forehead, nose, and chin.

Dermatologists call this the "T-zone". People should moisturise dry regions only and avoid moisturising greasy areas. Depending on how dry the skin is, a light gel moisturiser, a cream-based product, or an ointment may be used.

For those who shave, shave with a moisturising shaving cream. Also, shave in the same way that your hair grows. After each shave, rinse the razor. After 5-7 shaves, replace the blade.

If you have ingrown hairs, razor burn, or razor bumps, use a single- or double-blade razor and avoid pulling the skin during shaving.

Coloured Skin

Higher melanin levels in the skin can make the skin more prone to hyperpigmentation. Hyperpigmentation can occur as a result of pimples, a psoriasis patch, or a healed injury, certain drugs, products that cause skin irritation, hormone fluctuations, such as those seen during pregnancy and so on.

A doctor may refer to a hyperpigmented area as post-inflammatory hyperpigmentation if it is caused by pimples, injury, or psoriasis.

2

The Most Important Anti-Aging Ingredients

Before beginning an anti-aging skin care programme, look for these five anti-aging components in your favourite products.

Retinol

Retinol, a vitamin A derivative, is one of the most frequently used and examined compounds in skincare products. It is well-known for its several skin advantages, particularly in addressing aging indications and enhancing general skin texture and look. Here's a rundown of retinol's effects:

1. Anti-aging: Retinol is primarily used for its anti-aging properties, as it stimulates the production of collagen, a protein that provides firmness to the skin, making it more rigid while decreasing the appearance of fine lines and wrinkles. Retinol also helps to improve skin elasticity and smooth the skin's surface by stimulating collagen synthesis.

2. Acne treatment: By controlling oil production and boosting skin cell turnover, retinol can help clear pores and minimise acne outbreaks.

3. Skin texture and tone: It can smooth out skin texture and even out skin tone by removing hyper-pigmentation and dark patches.

4. Healing of sun damage: Retinol may aid in the healing of sun damage produced by ultraviolet (UV) radiation.

When using retinol in skincare, it is critical to follow the product's directions and begin with a lesser dose to allow the skin to acclimatise. When first starting retinol, some people might encounter skin irritation, redness, or flakiness, although these effects usually fade with regular use.

It's important to note that retinol might make your skin more susceptible to the sun, so use sunscreen every day if you're making use of retinol-based products to protect your skin from UV damage.

Apart from its aesthetic use, retinol is an essential component in our diet, found in foods such as liver, fish, dairy products, and certain fruits and vegetables, and it plays an important role in maintaining good vision, enhancing immunological function, and supporting cell growth and development.

Vitamin C

This antioxidant will safeguard your skin from free radicals as well as UV damage. When utilised in skincare regimes, vitamin C is a potent antioxidant that provides several advantages to the skin. As an antioxidant, it aids in the neutralisation of free radicals, which are unstable chemicals that can cause skin cell damage and premature ageing. Here are some of the ways Vitamin C can help with skincare:

1. Brightening and Balancing Skin Tone: Vitamin C can aid in the fading of dark spots, hyperpigmentation, and age spots, resulting in a more even and luminous complexion. It helps to lighten the skin by

inhibiting the formation of melanin, the pigment responsible for dark spots.

2. Collagen production: Vitamin C is required for collagen production, a protein that provides structure and elasticity to the skin. Vitamin C helps improve skin firmness and minimise the appearance of fine lines and wrinkles by promoting collagen formation.

3. Sun Protection: While Vitamin C is not a replacement for sunscreen, it can improve the efficiency of sunscreens and provide an additional layer of protection against dangerous UV rays. It can help restore some of the sun damage to the skin produced by UV light exposure.

4. Anti-inflammatory qualities: Anti-inflammatory qualities of vitamin C can help soothe and calm inflamed or

sensitive skin. It may be good for people who have rosacea or acne-prone skin.

Consider the following tips for including Vitamin C in your skincare routine:

- Choose the Right Product: Look for goods containing stable forms of Vitamin C, such as L-ascorbic acid, sodium ascorbyl phosphate, or ascorbyl palmitate. These kinds are more likely to retain their effectiveness and not deteriorate soon.

- Concentration: Products with 10% to 20% Vitamin C concentrations are often helpful without causing considerable discomfort. If you have sensitive skin, start with a lower concentration and progressively increase it if your skin tolerates it well.

- Storage: Vitamin C items are light, air, and heat sensitive, which can cause oxidation and impair their effectiveness.

Keep them in dark, closed containers away from direct sunlight.

- Time of Use: Apply vitamin C in the morning to help protect the skin from environmental harm throughout the day. However, if it works better for you, you can incorporate it into your bedtime regimen.

- Combination with additional Ingredients: To increase its potency, vitamin C can be mixed with additional antioxidants such as vitamin E and ferulic acid. Furthermore, it can be used in conjunction with other skincare compounds such as hyaluronic acid and retinol to create a full anti-aging regimen.

Before applying Vitamin C to your face, as with any new skincare product, perform a patch test to verify your skin does not react negatively. If you have any concerns or specific skin disorders, contact a dermatologist to identify the appropriate Vitamin C supplement and routine for your skin type.

AHAs (Alpha Hydroxy Acids)

To exfoliate and remove dead skin cells, alpha hydroxy acids such as glycolic and citric acid are utilised. Alpha Hydroxy Acids (AHAs) are a class of water-soluble acids known for their exfoliating and rejuvenating qualities in cosmetics. These acids come from a variety of natural sources, including fruits, milk, and sugarcane. AHAs operate by breaking down the links between dead skin cells on the skin's surface, allowing dull and damaged skin to be removed, revealing smoother, brighter, and more even-toned skin beneath. AHAs that are commonly utilised in skincare include:

- Glycolic Acid: Glycolic acid is derived from sugarcane and is one of the most commonly used AHAs. It has a small molecular size, which allows it to penetrate the skin deeply and effectively exfoliate. Glycolic acid is suitable for most skin types, especially those with concerns about dullness, fine lines, and uneven texture.

- Lactic Acid: Lactic acid is derived from milk and is known for its gentle exfoliating properties.

- Citric Acid: Citric acid, found in citrus fruits such as lemons and oranges, is a natural AHA with antioxidant characteristics. It can assist to brighten the skin and improve the general texture of the skin.

- Malic Acid: Another moderate AHA derived from apples, malic acid aids in exfoliating and rejuvenating the skin's surface.

- Tartaric Acid: Found in grapes, tartaric acid improves skin tone and texture while assisting other AHAs in exfoliating.

Here are some of the ways that AHAs help in skincare:

1. Exfoliation: AHAs promote gentle exfoliation, removing dead skin cells and which allows other skincare products to penetrate more effectively. Improves Skin Texture: AHAs can help smoother, softer skin and reduce the appearance of fine lines and wrinkles.

2. Evens Skin Tone: AHAs can help fade dark spots, hyperpigmentation, and sun

damage, resulting in a more even skin tone.

3. AHAs increase collagen synthesis, which aids in the improvement of skin suppleness and firmness.

4. AHAs improve product absorption by eliminating the top layer of dead skin cells, allowing serums and moisturisers to penetrate deeper into the skin.

AHAs should be used with caution because they can make the skin more susceptible to the sun. When using AHAs in your skincare routine, it is critical to apply sunscreen daily to protect the skin from UV damage. Additionally, begin with lesser AHA concentrations and gradually increase as your skin develops tolerance. Before beginning a new skincare routine with AHAs, contact a dermatologist if you have sensitive skin or any concerns.

Vitamin E

Vitamin E is a fat-soluble antioxidant that has various skin benefits when used in skincare products. It protects the skin from damage produced by free radicals, which are unstable chemicals that can cause premature aging and other skin problems. Here are some of the ways Vitamin E can help with skincare:

1. Vitamin E, as an antioxidant, helps neutralise free radicals, lowering oxidative stress and protecting the skin from environmental damage such as pollution and UV rays.

2. Moisturization: Vitamin E is a great moisturiser since it keeps the skin moisturised and prevents moisture loss. It

can increase the skin's ability to retain water, resulting in softer, more supple skin.

3. Vitamin E has anti-inflammatory properties, which can help heal and calm irritated or inflamed skin. Individuals suffering from eczema or psoriasis may benefit from it.

4. Wound Healing: Vitamin E promotes tissue repair and helps the skin's natural healing process. It may also help minimise the appearance of scars.

5. UV Protection Enhancement: While not a replacement for sunscreen, when taken with Vitamin C, Vitamin E can improve the efficacy of sunscreens and give additional UV protection.

6. Anti-Aging: The antioxidant properties of vitamin E can help protect against

premature ageing indications such as fine lines, wrinkles, and age spots.

Vitamin E is present in a variety of skincare products such as creams, serums, oils, and moisturisers. It is frequently used in concert with other antioxidants such as Vitamin C, as well as substances such as hyaluronic acid and retinol, to build comprehensive anti-aging and moisturising skincare routines.

Because some people are sensitive or allergic to Vitamin E, a patch test is required before using a new skincare product that includes this vitamin, especially if you have sensitive skin or have a previous history of allergies. Furthermore, because vitamin E is light and air sensitive, it is more stable and effective when stored in opaque or airtight packaging.

In conclusion, Vitamin E is an important element in skincare since it protects the skin from oxidative damage, moisturises it, and promotes general skin health. It is a versatile addition to skincare regimes that can work in tandem with other substances to address specific skin issues.

Collagen

Collagen is a protein found naturally in the skin that helps to preserve its structure, firmness, and suppleness. It is also known as the "fundamental component" of the skin. The body's production of collagen steadily diminishes as we age, resulting in fine lines, wrinkles, and sagging skin. As a result, collagen has grown in popularity as an ingredient in skincare products and treatments. Here are some examples of how collagen is utilised in skincare:

1. Collagen is widely used in anti-aging skincare products due to its ability to increase skin elasticity and firmness. It can help minimise the look of wrinkles and fine lines by increasing collagen in the skin, either topically or through treatments.

2. Hydration & Moisturization: Because collagen attracts and retains moisture, it is a beneficial component for hydrating the skin. It contributes to the preservation of the skin's natural moisture barrier, avoiding dryness and keeping the skin supple and soft.

3. Skin Texture Improvement: When applied topically, collagen can help enhance skin texture by making it smoother and more even.

4. Wound Healing and Scarring: Collagen is involved in the normal healing process of the skin. It can be used topically to aid wound healing and possibly minimise the appearance of scars.

5. Plumping and Volume: Collagen is used as a filler in some cosmetic operations to add volume to specific parts of the face, such as the lips or cheeks, to achieve plumper and more youthful appearance.

While collagen is good for the skin, the collagen molecules in most topical-use skincare products are too big to properly penetrate the skin's surface. As a result, the collagen component of these products may have a limited direct influence on boosting collagen levels in the skin. Instead, some skin care products contain chemicals like peptides, retinol, and Vitamin C that can boost the skin's natural collagen production. These chemicals have the potential to be more effective in stimulating long-term collagen formation and skin regeneration.

It is critical to speak with a skilled medical expert before undergoing collagen treatments or procedures such as collagen injections to evaluate the potential dangers, advantages, and suitability for individual skin conditions.

In conclusion, collagen is an important component of skin care since it helps improve skin elasticity, moisture, and texture. While topical collagen supplementation has certain advantages, increasing the skin's natural collagen production along with other substances may have a more significant and long-term influence on skin health and anti-aging efforts.

3

<u>Five Anti-Aging Face Tools to Include in Your Routine</u>

Skincare tools can also help firm and elevate the face, which can be beneficial for anti-aging. Discover five facial tools to incorporate into your routine below.

Jade Roller

A jade roller is a portable beauty product used in skincare routines that is noted for its skin-cooling and massaging properties. It is a little roller with one or two smooth, rounded jade stones connected to each end of the handle. Jade stones are typically constructed of real jade or other gemstones such as rose quartz.

Jade rollers have been used for centuries in traditional Chinese skincare practices and have recently gained appeal as part of modern cosmetic routines. Here's how jade rollers are commonly used.

How to Make Use of a Jade Roller:

- Preparation: Cleanse your face and apply your favourite serum, oil, or moisturiser to create some slip to the skin, allowing the roller to glide smoothly.

- Cooling Effect: Jade is naturally cool to the touch, which can help relax and depuff the skin. Some individuals like to chill the jade roller before using it to increase the cooling sensation.

- Facial Massage: Roll the jade roller in an outward and upward motion over different parts of your face. The smaller end is for more delicate areas like the under-eye area, while the larger end is for wider areas like the cheeks and forehead.

- Neck and Décolletage: For a relaxing massage, use the jade roller on your neck and décolletage.
- When rolling the jade roller, employ delicate pressure; too much pressure can cause skin discomfort.

Advantages of Using a Jade Roller:

1. **Lymphatic Drainage:** The jade roller's rolling motion may aid in lymphatic drainage, reducing puffiness around the face and increasing circulation.
2. **Reduced Puffiness:** The jade roller's cooling impact can help constrict blood vessels and reduce puffiness around the eyes and face.

3. **Relaxation and Stress Relief:** The jade roller's massaging effect can be calming and may help reduce tension and stress.

4. **Enhanced Product Absorption:** Pressing serums or moisturisers into the skin with a jade roller may aid improve product absorption.

While jade rollers can give a relaxing and calming sensation, their effects on the skin are quite moderate. They are not intended to be a replacement for medical-grade skincare products or treatments for specific skin conditions.

After each usage, simply wash your jade roller with gentle soap and water and wipe it dry. Hot water and harsh chemicals should be avoided as they can destroy the jade and its characteristics.

Overall, including a jade roller in your skincare routine may be a calming and delightful addition, delivering a little moment of self-care as well as potentially moderate skin benefits.

Gua Sha

Gua sha is an ancient Chinese medicinal procedure in which the skin is scraped using a smooth-edged tool made of jade, rose quartz, or other materials such as buffalo horn or earthenware. The phrase "gua sha" means "scraping sand" in Chinese, because it causes redness on the skin that looks like a sand rash. Gua sha has been utilised in traditional Chinese medicine for centuries for a variety of therapeutic objectives, including increasing blood circulation, decreasing inflammation, and relieving muscle tension.

Gua sha has gained popularity in the beauty and wellness sector in recent years as a facial treatment to improve skin health and attractiveness. Here's how gua sha is utilised.

How to use Gua Sha for Face massage:

- Prepare your face by cleansing it and applying facial oil or serum to create lubrication for the gua sha tool.

- Apply mild pressure while holding the gua sha instrument at a 15-degree angle to the skin. Scrape the tool gently upward and outward, following the curves of your face and neck.

- Order: Begin at the centre of your face and work your way outwards. Lighter strokes around the eyes and more firm pressure on the cheeks, jawline, and forehead are recommended.

Gua sha can be performed 2-3 times per week or as desired, but it is critical not to overdo it to avoid skin irritation.

Gua Sha Facial Massage May Have These Advantages:

1. Gua sha, like the jade roller, can assist improve lymphatic drainage, reducing puffiness and oedema in the face.

2. Circulation Stimulation: The scraping action of gua sha may help stimulate blood flow to the skin, providing a healthy complexion.

3. Tension Relief: Gently massaging the face and neck with a gua sha tool can help relieve muscle tension.

4. Improvements in circulation and lymphatic drainage may result in a brighter, more radiant complexion.

5. Product Absorption: Gua sha, like jade rolling, can improve the absorption of skincare products into the skin.

To avoid skin irritation or bruising, gua sha should be performed softly and without exerting undue pressure. People who have rosacea, dermatitis, or aggressive acne should avoid gua sha or visit a physician before using the method. Individual outcomes may vary, like with any cosmetic or skincare practice, and it is critical to be consistent and patient to observe the possible advantages of gua sha facial massage. If you're not sure how to incorporate gua sha into your practice, talk to a professional or an experienced practitioner who can advise you on proper procedures and usage.

Microcurrent Device

A handheld electronic beauty gadget that uses low-level electrical currents to stimulate and tone facial muscles is known as a microcurrent device. It is intended to stimulate the body's natural electrical currents, which are involved in muscle contraction and skin rigidity. Microcurrent devices have acquired appeal in the cosmetic business due to their ability to improve skin texture, reduce wrinkle appearance, and provide non-invasive facial toning.

Here's how microcurrent devices function,

- Microcurrent devices emit low-level electrical currents, often in the microampere range, which are very light and generally safe for the skin.

- Muscle Stimulation: When microcurrents are applied to the skin, they stimulate the underlying facial muscles, making them contract and tone. This is also known as "facial sculpting" or "facial lifting."

- Microcurrents may also aid enhance blood circulation, which can result in improved skin texture and a more luminous complexion.

- Product Absorption is Improved: The stimulation from the microcurrents can help with the absorption of skincare products used before or after the treatment.

Microcurrent Devices' Potential Benefits:

1. The fundamental advantage of microcurrent devices is their ability to raise and tone face muscles, resulting in a more sculpted and young appearance.

2. Reduced Fine Lines and Wrinkles: Increased muscle tone can help minimise the appearance of fine lines and wrinkles, especially on the forehead, around the eyes, and the lips.

3. Improved Skin Texture: Improved skin texture and a more even complexion may result from increased circulation and improved product absorption.

Microcurrent treatments are often non-invasive and painless, making them a popular alternative to more harsh facial procedures. While microcurrent devices can produce visible improvements, they are not a substitute for surgical face lifts or other medical cosmetic operations for more severe skin aging concerns. The effects of microcurrent treatments are frequently transient, and consistent use is usually required to maintain the results.

When utilising a microcurrent device, it is critical to carefully follow the manufacturer's recommendations and begin with lower intensity levels, gradually increasing as your skin adjusts to the treatment. Also, avoid utilising microcurrent devices over open wounds, irritated skin, or areas with metal implants because the electrical currents may be interfered with.

If you're thinking about introducing a microcurrent device into your skincare routine, go to a dermatologist or skincare professional first to make sure it's safe for your skin type and to learn the right practices for best results.

Dermaplaning

Dermaplaning is a cosmetic skincare process that exfoliates the top layer of skin, specifically the outermost layer of dead skin cells and vellus hair (also known as "peach fuzz"). This procedure is usually carried out by a licenced skincare specialist, such as an esthetician or a dermatologist.

During a dermaplaning session, the practitioner softly scrapes across the skin's surface at a 45-degree angle with a sterile medical scalpel. This procedure aids in the removal of dead skin cells, debris, oil, and other impurities from the skin, leaving it smoother, softer, and more luminous.

Dermaplaning has several major advantages, including:

- Improved skin texture: Dermaplaning can help reveal fresher, smoother skin beneath by eliminating the outer layer of dead skin cells.

- Product absorption is improved after dermaplaning because skincare products may penetrate the skin more efficiently, maximising their effects.

- Exfoliation can assist to minimise the appearance of fine lines and wrinkles and give the skin a more youthful appearance.

- Even skin tone: Dermaplaning can help to get a more even complexion by fading hyperpigmentation or dark patches.

- Temporary vellus hair removal: The technique can also eliminate fine, light-coloured facial hair, allowing for a smoother makeup application and a brighter appearance.

It is critical to highlight that dermaplaning is a non-invasive procedure that is appropriate for most skin types. It is not, however, recommended for people who have active acne or certain skin diseases. If you're thinking about getting dermaplaning, talk to a qualified skincare specialist first to see if it's right for your skin type and any specific concerns you may have. Furthermore, it is critical to protect your skin from sun exposure following the surgery and to follow the post-treatment care instructions advised by the practitioner.

Facial Cleansing Brush

A facial cleansing brush is a portable electronic device that helps scrub the skin more effectively than traditional manual methods. A motorised brush head with soft bristles or silicone nodes that rotate or vibrate to wash the skin is typical. A facial washing brush operates as follows:

- Wet your skin before using the brush, and then put a tiny bit of facial cleanser on the brush head or straight on your face.

- Turn on the device: Most facial washing brushes have numerous speed settings, allowing you to select the level of intensity that is appropriate for your skin type and preferences.

- Gently move the brush around your face in circular strokes using little pressure. Begin in the centre and work your way outward, paying special attention to the forehead, cheeks, nose, and chin. Avoid touching the delicate areas around your eyes.

- Cleanse for the specified period: The manufacturer normally specifies a time for cleansing. It is usually between one and two minutes.

- After cleansing, properly rinse your face with water to eliminate the cleanser and pollutants from your skin.

Note the following points;

a) Concerning your skin type and sensitivity, you may only need to use the brush once or twice a day. Excessive use may cause discomfort.

b) Replacement: To preserve hygiene and efficacy, the brush head should be replaced regularly, usually every few months.

c) Sensitive skin: If you have sensitive skin, you should use a brush with softer bristles or a silicone brush, which is kinder on the skin.

d) Compatibility with your skincare products: Some facial washing brushes may perform better with certain cleansers. Always follow the manufacturer's instructions.

e) Consider your skin type and any skin issues you may have before using a facial washing brush. It is recommended to begin with a lesser speed and gradually raise it if necessary. If you develop any irritation or unpleasant reactions, stop using the product and see a dermatologist.

4

<u>Ten Anti-aging Skincare Recommendations</u>

Incorporate these ten anti-aging skin care tips into your routine to reduce the appearance of fine lines and wrinkles, as well as promote collagen and hydration.

01.Cleanse with a cream cleanser.

Washing with a cream cleanser is a common component in the skincare process. Cream cleansers are mild and moisturising, making them ideal for a variety of skin types, particularly dry or sensitive skin. If you have noticeably aging skin, use a nourishing cream cleanser rather than a foamy one, which can be harsh for a sensitive face. Skin loses moisture, nutrients, and natural oils as it ages, resulting in skin that appears and feels dry. A cream cleanser can help refill moisture on the skin's surface for a more youthful appearance. Here's a general guide to using a cream cleanser on your face:

1. **Begin with clean hands:** Before touching your face, make sure your hands are free of dirt and bacteria.

2. **Wet your face:** To prepare your skin for cleansing, splash it with lukewarm water.

3. **Apply the cream cleanser:** Using gentle, circular strokes, apply a little amount of the cream cleanser to your face. Concentrate on areas that have makeup, grime, or excess oil.

4. **Massage gently:** For around 1-2 minutes, massage the cream cleanser into your skin with your fingertips. This aids in the

removal of pollutants and improves blood circulation.

5. **Rinse:** After rubbing, properly rinse your face with lukewarm water to eliminate all of the cleansers. Hot water should be avoided since it is too harsh on the skin.

6. **Dry your face:** After cleansing, pat your face dry gently with a clean, soft cloth. Avoid rubbing your skin as this can irritate it.

7. **Apply moisturiser after cleansing:** Because cream cleansers are often moisturising, you may not require an extra moisturiser immediately after cleansing. If your skin still feels dry, use a lightweight, non-comedogenic moisturiser.

Use a cream cleanser twice a day, once in the morning and once in the evening, or alter the frequency based on the needs of your skin. Some people may prefer to use it solely in the evening to remove makeup and pollutants that have accumulated over the day.

Remember that everyone's skin is unique, so choose items that are appropriate for your skin type. If you have any specific skin concerns or conditions, it's always a good idea to seek personalised guidance from a dermatologist.

02. Exfoliate once a week

Exfoliating your skin has numerous benefits, including eliminating dead skin cells and whitening skin, making it a crucial part of an anti-aging skincare routine. Exfoliating your skin weekly is a great addition to your skincare routine because it helps to remove dead skin cells and promote a smoother, more radiant complexion. However, the frequency of exfoliation can vary depending on your skin type and the type of exfoliator you're using. Here's a general guide to weekly exfoliation:

Select the best exfoliator: Physical exfoliators, which contain microscopic particles that physically brush away dead skin cells, and chemical exfoliators, which employ acids to dissolve dead skin cells, are the two main types of exfoliators. You may prefer one over the other depending on your skin type and sensitivity.

1. **Cleanse your face:** Before exfoliating, begin with a gentle cleanser to remove any makeup, debris, or pollutants.

2. **Usage:** If you're using a physical exfoliator, wet your face slightly before applying a little amount of the product. Use gentle, circular strokes to massage it into your skin. If you're using a chemical exfoliator, make sure you know how to use it correctly. Avoid severe scrubbing or

excessive pressure while using a physical or chemical exfoliant, as this might irritate your skin. Allow the exfoliator to do its work.

3. **Rinse:** After exfoliating, properly rinse your face with lukewarm water until all of the exfoliant has been removed.

4. **Moisturise:** Because exfoliation might temporarily make your skin more sensitive, it's critical to use a moisturiser afterwards to keep your skin hydrated and protected.

Exfoliating once a week is sufficient for most people. If you have sensitive or dry skin, you should exfoliate less frequently, perhaps every 10-14 days. If you have oily or acne-prone skin, you may be able to exfoliate more frequently, but be careful not to overdo it, as this might cause discomfort.

Excessive exfoliation can rob your skin of its natural oils and cause discomfort. Reduce the frequency of exfoliation or switch to a lighter exfoliator if you detect any redness, excessive dryness, or irritation after exfoliating.

Always pay attention to your skin and adapt your exfoliating routine as needed. If you're not sure which exfoliant is ideal for your skin type or have specific skin concerns, consult a dermatologist for personalised advice.

03. Use a facial serum.

Facial serums are lightweight skincare products with high active ingredient concentrations. They are intended to address specific skin issues and give a more potent and intensive treatment than standard moisturisers. Serums are often thin and quickly absorbed by the skin, delivering active chemicals deep into the epidermis.

There are several varieties of face serums on the market, each designed to target a specific skin condition, such as:

- **Hydrating serums:** These serums are designed to provide and maintain moisture in the skin, making them ideal for dry or dehydrated skin.
- **Anti-aging serums**: These serums frequently contain retinol, vitamin C, peptides, and antioxidants to minimise fine lines and wrinkles and enhance skin elasticity.
- **Brightening serums:** These serums target dark spots, hyperpigmentation, and uneven skin tone using ingredients like

vitamin C, niacinamide, and alpha hydroxy acids (AHAs).

- Serums with acne-fighting chemicals such as salicylic acid or benzoyl peroxide can help decrease oil production, clear pores, and reduce acne outbreaks.

- **Soothing serums:** These serums are intended to soothe and minimise redness and irritation, and they frequently contain substances such as aloe vera, chamomile, or green tea extracts.

When using a face serum, use the proper amount, usually a few drops, and gently massage it into the skin in upward motions.

After the serum has been absorbed, apply your regular moisturiser to lock in the benefits. Check the product's instructions for particular usage recommendations, since some serums can be used once or twice a day, but others are more concentrated and require less frequent application.

Patch-testing any new serum before applying it to your entire face is also essential, especially if you have sensitive skin or are trying a new product for the first time. If you have any questions about how to use a facial serum or which one is best for your skin type, seek personalised guidance from a dermatologist or skincare professional.

04. Use a specialised eye cream.

Eye creams are skincare treatments that are specifically created for sensitive skin around the eyes. This area's skin is thinner and more sensitive than the rest of the face, leaving it more prone to dryness, fine wrinkles, and puffiness. Eye creams often contain a combination of active substances that address specific eye issues, such as:

- **Moisturising:** Hydrating substances such as hyaluronic acid, glycerin, and ceramides are commonly found in eye creams to help maintain the moisture barrier of the skin and prevent dryness and dehydration.

- **Anti-aging:** Some eye creams comprise ingredients like retinol, peptides, and vitamin C to address fine lines, wrinkles, and loss of elasticity around the eyes.

- **Brightening:** Eye creams with ingredients like vitamin C, niacinamide, and kojic acid can help minimise dark circles and brighten the under-eye area. Firming: Eye creams may contain collagen and elastin to improve the skin's firmness and elasticity.

Here are some general guidelines for using eye cream:

1. **Use twice a day:** For best results, use the eye cream in both your morning and nightly skincare routines.

2. **Use Regularly:** Regular and continuous use of eye cream can result in better benefits over time.

3. When applying the lotion, avoid twisting or pulling at the delicate skin around your eyes.

4. Keep the eye cream away from the lash line to prevent the product from getting into the eyes.

5. **Avoid using too much product:** With eye creams, a little goes a long way, so use carefully to avoid overloading the delicate eye area.

As with any skincare product, selecting an eye cream that addresses your individual needs and skin type is critical. If you have any underlying eye diseases or concerns, you should get personalised guidance from a dermatologist or ophthalmologist.

05. Moisturise with consideration for your skin type.

Moisturising is an important component in any skincare routine, and selecting the proper moisturiser for your skin type may make a big difference in keeping your skin healthy and balanced. Here's a general guide to moisturising for different skin types:

Normal Skin Type:

Normal skin is well-balanced, with sufficient sebum production and few issues. To keep the skin's natural moisture without making it oily, use a lightweight, non-greasy moisturiser.

Dry Skin:

Dry skin is dehydrated and may feel tight or flaky. To replace moisture and improve skin barrier function, use a thick, creamy moisturiser containing hydrating ingredients such as hyaluronic acid, glycerin, or ceramides.

Oily Skin:

Excess sebum is produced by oily skin, resulting in a glossy appearance and the possibility of acne breakouts. Choose a lightweight, oil-free, non-comedogenic moisturiser that will not clog pores. To regulate oil and decrease acne, look for substances like niacinamide or salicylic acid.

Combination Skin Type:

Combination skin is a blend of several skin types, with oily T-zone and normal to dry cheeks.

Apply a lightweight, non-greasy moisturiser to the driest regions of your face, avoiding heavy application in the T-zone.

Sensitive Skin:

Sensitive skin is prone to redness and reactions and is easily irritated. Look for a fragrance-free moisturiser that contains soothing ingredients such as aloe vera, chamomile, or oat extracts.

Acne-prone Skin:

Acne-prone skin demands a moisturiser that will not worsen outbreaks and may aid in oil control. To treat acne, use an oil-free, non-comedogenic moisturiser containing substances such as tea tree oil or salicylic acid.

Matured Skin:

Anti-aging chemicals that target fine lines and elasticity loss may benefit mature skin. To encourage skin regeneration, use a moisturiser containing retinol, peptides, or antioxidants.

Remember that everyone's skin concerns are different, so pay attention to how your skin reacts to different moisturisers. If you have specific skin disorders or concerns, you should always contact a dermatologist or skincare professional to determine the best moisturiser for your skin type. Furthermore, patch testing any new product is recommended, especially if you have sensitive or reactive skin.

06. Use a facial oil

Facial oils are skincare products that contain various plant-based or natural oils that offer nourishing and moisturising benefits to the skin. These oils are typically lightweight and quickly absorbed, making them suitable for different skin types, including dry, oily, combination, and sensitive skin. The most common types include,

- **Rosehip Oil:** Rosehip oil, which is high in vitamins, antioxidants, and vital fatty acids, improves skin texture, reduces the appearance of scars and fine lines, and promotes skin regeneration.

- **Argan Oil:** Because of its high vitamin E concentration, argan oil moisturises and nourishes the skin, making it an excellent choice for dry and older skin.

- **Marula Oil:** Rich in antioxidants, marula oil protects the skin from environmental damage and is ideal for all skin types due to its lightweight texture.

- **Grapeseed Oil:** Non-comedogenic and high in linoleic acid, grapeseed oil is ideal for oily and acne-prone skin because it balances oil production and does not clog pores.

- **Chamomile Oil:** Chamomile oil has calming effects that can help calm irritated or sensitive skin and minimise redness.
- **Tea Tree Oil:** Known for its antimicrobial characteristics, tea tree oil can help reduce blemishes and irritation in acne-prone skin.

A little goes a long way when it comes to face oil. After cleansing and toning, add a few drops of the oil to your fingertips and gently press or massage it into your skin before applying moisturiser. Apply the face oil last if you're using other skincare products, such as serums or treatments, to lock in the benefits of the other products.

As with any new skincare product, patch-test the oil on a small area of your skin to check for any negative reactions, especially if you have sensitive skin or are using a new oil for the first time. Consult a dermatologist or skincare specialist if you have specific skin concerns or conditions to find the best face oil for you.

07. Apply SPF every day.

Sun Protection Factor (SPF) is a measure of how well a sunscreen or sunblock shields the skin from the harmful effects of ultraviolet (UV) radiation from the sun. SPF is an important component of sun protection since it helps to prevent sunburn, premature aging, and skin cancer.

When you apply sunscreen with a specified SPF number, it indicates how much longer you can stay in the sun without getting burned than if you don't wear any sunscreen at all. As an example:

- SPF 15: Offers approximately 15 times the protection against sunburn as no sunscreen. It is effective at blocking 93% of UVB rays.

- SPF 30: Provides approximately 30 times the protection against sunburn as no sunscreen. It is effective at blocking 97% of UVB rays.

- SPF 50: Offers approximately 50 times the protection against sunburn as no sunscreen. It blocks approximately 98% of UVB radiation.

It's crucial to remember that no sunscreen can offer complete protection from the sun's rays. As a result, it's always a good idea to take additional sun protection precautions, such as seeking shade during peak sun hours (about 10 a.m. to 4 p.m.), wearing protective clothes, and wearing sunglasses to protect your eyes.

Here are some things to remember when applying sunscreen:

1. **Apply liberally:** Use enough sunscreen to cover all exposed regions of your skin, including your ears, the back of your neck, and the tips of your feet.

2. **Re-apply sunscreen frequently:** Because sunscreen effectiveness fades over time, reapply every two hours, or more frequently if you're swimming or sweating.

3. **Water-resistant sunscreen:** If you're going to be swimming or sweating, use a water-resistant sunscreen, but remember to reapply afterwards.

4. **Broad-spectrum protection:** Look for sunscreens labelled "broad-spectrum," which block both UVA and UVB rays.

5. **Examine expiration dates:** Because sunscreens have an expiration date, be sure your product is still functional before applying it.

6. **Sunscreen for all skin types:** Regardless of skin colour or ethnicity, sunscreen is required for all skin types.

Remember that sun protection is essential for general skin health and reducing the risk of UV damage, premature aging, and skin cancer. If you have specific concerns regarding sun protection or skincare, always visit a dermatologist.

08. Gently Remove Makeup

It is critical to remove makeup gently to avoid irritating or harming your skin, especially the delicate areas around your eyes. Here are some ways for removing makeup effectively and gently:

1. Use a gentle makeup remover: Select a makeup remover that is made exclusively for your skin type. Choose a fragrance-free, light product for sensitive skin.

2. If you wear thick makeup or waterproof products, consider using an oil-based cleanser first to break down the makeup. Oils can effectively remove makeup without rough rubbing.

3. The skin around the eyes is fragile and prone to wrinkles. When removing eye makeup, use a gentle touch. Apply the makeup remover to a cotton pad and gently press it against the closed eye for a few seconds to allow the makeup to dissolve before wiping it away gently.

4. Hot water can be drying and unpleasant to the skin, so avoid using it. Instead, cleanse your face with lukewarm water.

5. Avoid using rough or abrasive materials that might cause friction and irritation by utilising soft cotton pads or a microfiber towel. Instead, gently remove makeup with delicate cotton pads or a microfiber cloth.

6. Pat, not rub: Instead of forcefully rubbing off makeup, employ a soft patting motion. Patting helps to reduce needless skin tugging.

7. After using a makeup remover or oil cleanser, thoroughly rinse your face with lukewarm water to remove any residue.

8. Follow with a gentle cleanser: To ensure that your face is completely clean, use a

gentle, water-based cleanser to remove any remaining makeup and pollutants.

9. Consider the items you use: If you have sensitive skin or specific skin concerns, choose makeup removers free of harsh chemicals, alcohol, and smell.

10. After cleansing, moisturise with a moisturiser appropriate for your skin type to keep your skin moisturised and balanced.

You can maintain the health of your skin and avoid irritation or injury by being gentle and mindful during the makeup removal procedure.

09. At bedtime, apply a wrinkle cream.

Using a wrinkle cream at night can be a helpful addition to your skincare routine, especially if the look of fine lines and wrinkles is your primary concern. Because your skin is more responsive to active substances during the restorative sleep period, applying skincare products at night is great.

Here are some suggestions for including a wrinkle treatment in your evening skincare routine:

1. Start by cleaning your face to remove any makeup, dirt, or impurities that have gathered throughout the day. A clean canvas allows the wrinkle cream to penetrate deeper into the skin.

2. Apply the wrinkle cream: Apply a small amount of wrinkle cream (typically a pea-sized amount) to your face and neck. Concentrate on wrinkle-prone areas such as the forehead, around the eyes, and the mouth.

3. Massage it in: Massage the cream into your skin with gentle upward strokes.

Avoid pushing or tugging on the skin surrounding the delicate eye area.

4. Allow it to absorb: Allow the wrinkle cream to thoroughly seep into your skin before applying any other products. This could take some time.

5. Apply a moisturiser (optional): Depending on the formulation of your wrinkle cream, you may or may not need to apply a moisturiser afterwards. Moisturising elements are already present in several wrinkle creams. If your skin still feels dry after the wrinkle cream has been absorbed, use a second moisturiser.

6. Use the wrinkle cream frequently as part of your bedtime skincare routine for the best effects. It may take some time for wrinkles to disappear, so be patient and stick to the regimen.

7. Wear sunscreen during the day: Some wrinkle creams have components that can make your skin more sun sensitive. Use broad-spectrum sunscreen with an acceptable SPF during the day to protect your skin from UV damage.

Keep in mind that many wrinkle creams contain different active components, such as retinol, peptides, hyaluronic acid, or antioxidants. Choose a product that addresses your skin concerns and demands. Perform a patch test before applying the wrinkle cream to your complete face if you have sensitive skin or are trying a new product.

10. Sleep on a silk pillowcase

Sleeping on a silk pillowcase can provide several potential benefits for your skin and hair. Here are some of the benefits of using a silk pillowcase:

1. Reduced friction: Unlike cotton or other fabrics, silk has a smooth surface that creates less friction against your skin. This can help prevent sleep lines and creases on your face, which may contribute to premature ageing over time.

2. Maintaining moisture balance: Because silk is less absorbent than cotton, it can aid in the retention of natural moisture in your skin and hair as you sleep. This is especially good for people who have dry skin or hair.

3. Hair benefits: Using a silk pillowcase while sleeping might help prevent frizz and breakage. Silk's smooth surface allows your hair to slide effortlessly, eliminating the possibility of tangling or damage.

4. Silk is inherently hypoallergenic and resistant to dust mites and other allergens, making it a good choice for allergy sufferers.

5. Temperature regulation: Silk is a breathable fabric that can aid in the regulation of body temperature while sleeping, resulting in a comfortable and cool resting surface.

While silk pillowcases provide many advantages, it is crucial to note that they will not resolve all skin and hair issues on their own. A regular skincare routine, a good diet, and staying hydrated are all important for general skin health. When opting for a silk pillowcase, aim for one made of high-quality, pure silk. Blends with synthetic materials should be avoided because they may not deliver the same benefits as pure silk.

People's experiences may differ, and some people may not notice a substantial change when switching to a silk pillowcase. However, many users report enhanced comfort, and skin and hair advantages after using silk pillowcases regularly. Remember that, while silk pillowcases might provide benefits, they are only one component of a total skin care and hair care regimen.

5

<u>Age-tailored Skincare Routine for Juniors</u>

Our skin is constantly maturing, yet what you put on it in your 20s may be very different from what your skin requires in your 40s. Certain steps and their basics may remain constant, but the components and aims are likely to change. Follow these age-appropriate skincare routines for anti-aging results.

Anti-aging Skincare Routine for your Twenties

1. Cleanse: Every routine should begin with a face wash. Cleansing is vital because it removes debris, oil, and makeup from your skin. Here are a few recommendations for a thorough skincare cleansing routine:

- Choose the Right Cleanser: Choose a cleanser that is appropriate for your skin type. Consider using a gel-based or foamy cleanser to help reduce excess oil if you have oily skin. Choose a creamy or lotion-based cleanser that is mild and nourishing for dry or sensitive skin. Cleansers containing harsh compounds, such as sulphates, should be avoided since they can strip the skin of its natural oils.
- Wash Your Face Twice a Day: Cleanse your face twice a day, ideally in the

morning and evening. Cleansing in the morning helps eliminate any oils and pollutants that have accumulated overnight. It is beneficial to remove makeup, pollution, and debris from the day in the evening.

- Use Lukewarm Water: Before applying the cleanser, moisten your face with lukewarm water. Hot water can dehydrate the skin, while cold water may not efficiently remove debris and oils.

- Apply the cleanser to your damp face and gently massage it in circular strokes. Be gentle with your skin; cleaning too hard can cause irritation.

- Pay Attention to the T-Zone: If you have combination skin (oily T-zone and dry cheeks), concentrate your cleansing efforts on the T-zone (forehead, nose, and chin).

- Thoroughly rinse: Make sure to properly rinse off the cleanser, leaving no residue behind.

- After cleansing, wipe dry your face with a clean cloth. Avoid excessively rubbing your skin, as this might create irritation.

2. Treat Spots: For any skin issues, such as acne, hyperpigmentation, or dark spots, use a spot treatment or serum. Directly apply over-the-counter spot treatments comprising benzoyl peroxide, salicylic acid, or tea tree oil to the afflicted areas. These can aid in the reduction of inflammation and the killing of microorganisms.

3. Apply Eye Cream: Because the skin around your eyes is so fragile, applying an

eye cream or serum in your twenties can be beneficial.

4. Moisturize: Moisturiser is also an important step, regardless of your age or skin type, because your skin needs to be rehydrated after cleansing to keep the protective barrier on your skin strong and healthy.

5. Apply SPF: Sunscreen should be used as the final step in your skincare process, and then you can proceed to your makeup routine or go out for the day. Wear sunscreen with an SPF of at least 30, especially on cloudy days, and reapply every two hours if you're outside. Wearing a broad-brimmed hat and sunglasses can also help protect your face from UV rays.

Anti-aging Skin Care Routine for Your Thirties

Your skincare routine in your 30s will be equivalent to that of your 20s, with the addition of an exfoliation step to remove dead skin cells.

1. Cleanse: Your cleanser of choice can remain the same as long as you continue to wash your face twice a day.
2. Exfoliate: Cell turnover slows as you get older, thus exfoliation is critical. Remove dead skin cells with an exfoliating serum and say goodbye to dry, dull skin.
3. Apply moisturiser: Your skin may demand more hydration as it ages. Look for a moisturiser that contains components like hyaluronic acid, glycerin, and ceramides

to seal in moisture and keep your skin looking smooth and plump.

4. Add Retinol to your Routine: Retinol is a powerful type of vitamin A that can help enhance collagen formation, promote cell turnover, and minimise the appearance of fine lines and wrinkles. To avoid irritation, begin with a lesser concentration and gradually increase usage.

5. Eye Cream: Eye cream is still necessary, and you should apply it under the eyes to the temples. Tap any excess product in with your fingertips, then wait five minutes for the eye product to soak before moisturising.

6. Use SPF: Sunscreen should be a part of your daily routine by now, but if it isn't, there's no better time to start. Use a

broad-spectrum sunscreen with an SPF of 30 or higher every day, rain or shine.

7. Consider the following peptide-based products: Peptides are amino acid molecules that aid in collagen formation and skin firmness. Look for solutions that contain peptides to target specific areas with aging indications.

8. Use targeted treatments: To protect your skin from free radicals and environmental damage, incorporate products containing antioxidants such as vitamin C, resveratrol, or green tea extract.

9. Don't neglect your neck and décolletage: Extend your skincare routine to include your neck and chest, as these areas can also show signs of aging, apply sunscreen and moisturiser to these regions.

10. Hydrate and nurture your skin from within: Continue to drink lots of water and eat a balanced diet rich in skin-supporting nutrients such as vitamins A, C, E, and omega-3 fatty acids.

11. Avoid prolonged screen time: Blue light emitted by electronic gadgets has been linked to premature aging. To reduce the influence of blue light, consider wearing blue light filters or taking breaks from screens.

12. Professional treatments: To address specific skin issues and improve collagen formation, consider using professional treatments such as chemical peels, microdermabrasion, or laser therapy.

13. Minimise stress and get enough sleep: Because chronic stress can contribute to accelerated ageing, use stress-reduction

measures and make sure you receive enough restorative sleep.

Anti-Aging Skincare Routine for Your Forties

Because your skin may become drier as you age, an anti-aging skincare routine in your 40s should focus on replenishing moisture.

1. Cleanse: Your cleanser may be as moisturising and nourishing as your moisturiser since it employs restorative oils to cleanse your skin while gently yet effectively removing traces of makeup.

2. Make use of a moisturising serum: Add a moisturising serum to your anti-aging routine to ensure your skin is as nourished as possible. Look for hyaluronic acid as an

anti-aging component because it works with your skin's natural moisture to nourish and moisturise it.

3. Use Eye Cream: Eye cream helps keep your region hydrated and reduces the look of fine wrinkles and crow's feet. In your 40s, you can begin using eye cream in both your morning and evening regimens.

4. Apply moisturiser: As previously said, moisturiser is as necessary as ever. Choose a richer, thicker moisturiser, especially during dry seasons such as winter.

5. Continue to use sunscreen: Sunscreen is essential for preventing more damage and protecting your skin from dangerous UV rays. Apply a broad-spectrum sunscreen with an SPF of 30 or higher every day, and reapply as needed.

6. Retinol is your ally: In your 40s, retinol or prescribed retinoids can considerably benefit your skin. These products aid in the stimulation of collagen formation, the reduction of fine lines and wrinkles, and the improvement of skin texture.

7. Include the following growth ingredients in your daily routine: Proteins that encourage cell growth and collagen formation are known as growth factors. Look for products that contain growth elements to improve skin elasticity and firmness.

8. Hydration is essential: As your skin dries out, choose richer, more emollient moisturisers that provide deep hydration. Products containing hyaluronic acid can help maintain moisture and improve skin texture.

9. Manage stress and prioritise sleep: Stress and lack of sleep can both contribute to skin aging, so use stress-reduction tactics and get enough rest.

10. Consider the following professional treatments: Microdermabrasion, chemical peels, dermal fillers, and laser therapy are among the treatments that can help address specific difficulties and rejuvenate your skin.

11. Pay attention to your neck and hands: Extend your skincare routine to your neck and hands, as they might exhibit indications of aging as well. Regularly apply sunscreen and moisturiser to these areas.

12. Eat a skin-friendly diet: To nourish your skin from within, eat a balanced diet rich in fruits, vegetables, and healthy fats.

www.ingramcontent.com/pod-product-compliance
Lightning Source LLC
Chambersburg PA
CBHW060950260726
48661CB00005B/1826